THE OBSERVER

INNER HEALTH GAUGE
Non-attachment vs Hording

UNHINDERED
- Active
- Vulnerable
- Curious
- Alert
- Open-minded
- Observant
- Independent
- Excited
- Connected to my Heart

AVERAGE
- Arguing
- Cynical
- Preoccupied w Complicated Ideas
- Detached from Physical World & Heart
- High-Strung

UNHEALTHY
- Reclusive
- Unstable
- Phobic
- Rejecting Others
- Unable to Label Emotions
- Obsessed w Ideas
- Hording

Browse this gauge occasionally to assess whether your thoughts and habits are moving you more toward a place of fullness and non-attachment to things, or more toward the feeling of scarcity (leading to hording and phobias.)

Good questions to ask as you scan this gauge are:

What zone do I generally live in?

If it's not the healthiest zone, what changes do I need to make so I can take steps towards becoming a more emotionally healthy person?

There is so much knowledge to gain, but also, knowledge to use! And that may require knowing when to surface from observing and activate your knowledge...and share it with others.

Enter, the Observer.

Your mind is an incredible place, and there are people who value you and want to be involved in your life and thought processes. We hope the Observer will help you create healthy focuses and boundaries so you spend just as much time experiencing the world as you do observing it!

So...what do you want to explore and interact with today?

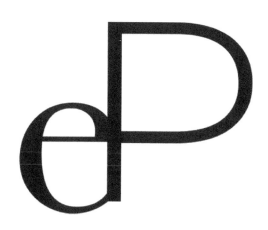

MONTH:

MONDAY	TUESDAY	WEDNESDAY	THURSDAY	FRIDAY	SATURDAY	SUNDAY

MONTH:

MONDAY	TUESDAY	WEDNESDAY	THURSDAY	FRIDAY	SATURDAY	SUNDAY

MONTH:

MONDAY	TUESDAY	WEDNESDAY	THURSDAY	FRIDAY	SATURDAY	SUNDAY

EXAMPLE PAGE

I DON'T NEED TO HAVE **ALL THE ANSWERS** TO JOIN THE **CONVERSATION**

TODAY'S DATE October 30th   **TODAY'S** GOAL Master Guitar HW

TODAY'S EXPLORATIONS	GIVES ENERGY	NEUTRAL	TAKES ENERGY
6am Breakfast	X		
7am			
8am			
9am			
10am			
11am			
12pm			
1pm Guitar lessons	X		
2pm			
3pm Work			X
4pm			
5pm			
6pm			
7pm			

TASKS	
Groceries	X
New Guitar strings	X
Research MAC repair	

MUST DO THIS WEEK

- Meal plan
- Finish LAB project

> It's okay if I'm not hitting all of these every season of life, but is there one I've been neglecting for awhile now? How is that going to effect my life long-term?

WHOLE-SELF CHECKLIST

- ☐ EXERCISE
- ☒ MEAL PLAN
- ☒ ALONE TIME
- ☐ SPIRITUAL INPUT
- ☐ SCHEDULED TIME TO PROCESS AN EXPERIENCE/FEELING

What is one step I can take to better my health?
I can clean out my garage and give some of the stuff I don't use consistently away.

Have I put up any walls? Is there anyone I need to forgive?
Julia hurt me...but she's been a good friend overall...I should call her.

What luxury can I give myself permission to enjoy today?
I'm going to get a good latte instead of 7-11 coffee today, because I DO have the money— I'm not in scarcity— and I'm worth it.

TOPIC	FORMAT	SOURCE
Birds	Podcast	Birder Life ep2

FAVORITE FACT:

The western bluebird has two broods per year!

> Use this space to record a topic you researched today/yesterday and your favorite takeaway!

I DON'T NEED TO HAVE **ALL THE ANSWERS** TO JOIN THE **CONVERSATION**

TODAY'S DATE **TODAY'S** GOAL

TODAY'S EXPLORATIONS	GIVES ENERGY	NEUTRAL	TAKES ENERGY	**T A S K S**

MUST DO THIS WEEK

What is one step I can take to better my health?

Have I put up any walls? Is there anyone I need to forgive?

What luxury can I give myself permission to enjoy today?

WHOLE-SELF
C H E C K L I S T
- EXERCISE
- MEAL PLAN
- ALONE TIME
- SPIRITUAL INPUT
- SCHEDULED TIME TO PROCESS AN EXPERIENCE/FEELING

TOPIC	FORMAT	SOURCE

FAVORITE FACT:

I DON'T NEED TO HAVE **ALL THE ANSWERS** TO JOIN THE **CONVERSATION**

TODAY'S DATE | **TODAY'S** GOAL

TODAY'S EXPLORATIONS	GIVES ENERGY	NEUTRAL	TAKES ENERGY	**T A S K S**

MUST DO THIS WEEK

WHOLE-SELF CHECKLIST
- EXERCISE
- MEAL PLAN
- ALONE TIME
- SPIRITUAL INPUT
- SCHEDULED TIME TO PROCESS AN EXPERIENCE/FEELING

What is one step I can take to better my health?

Have I put up any walls? Is there anyone I need to forgive?

What luxury can I give myself permission to enjoy today?

TOPIC	FORMAT	SOURCE

FAVORITE FACT:

I DON'T NEED TO HAVE **ALL THE ANSWERS** TO JOIN THE **CONVERSATION**

TODAY'S DATE **TODAY'S** GOAL

TODAY'S EXPLORATIONS	GIVES ENERGY	NEUTRAL	TAKES ENERGY	**T A S K S**

MUST DO THIS WEEK

What is one step I can take to better my health?

Have I put up any walls? Is there anyone I need to forgive?

What luxury can I give myself permission to enjoy today?

WHOLE-SELF CHECKLIST
- EXERCISE
- MEAL PLAN
- ALONE TIME
- SPIRITUAL INPUT
- SCHEDULED TIME TO PROCESS AN EXPERIENCE/FEELING

TOPIC	FORMAT	SOURCE

FAVORITE FACT:

I DON'T NEED TO HAVE **ALL THE ANSWERS** TO JOIN THE **CONVERSATION**

TODAY'S DATE

TODAY'S GOAL

TODAY'S EXPLORATIONS	GIVES ENERGY	NEUTRAL	TAKES ENERGY

T A S K S

MUST DO THIS WEEK

What is one step I can take to better my health?

Have I put up any walls? Is there anyone I need to forgive?

What luxury can I give myself permission to enjoy today?

WHOLE-SELF CHECKLIST
- EXERCISE
- MEAL PLAN
- ALONE TIME
- SPIRITUAL INPUT
- SCHEDULED TIME TO PROCESS AN EXPERIENCE/FEELING

TOPIC	FORMAT	SOURCE

FAVORITE FACT:

I DON'T NEED TO HAVE **ALL THE ANSWERS** TO JOIN THE **CONVERSATION**

TODAY'S DATE

TODAY'S GOAL

TODAY'S EXPLORATIONS	GIVES ENERGY	NEUTRAL	TAKES ENERGY	**T A S K S**

MUST DO THIS WEEK

What is one step I can take to better my health?

Have I put up any walls? Is there anyone I need to forgive?

What luxury can I give myself permission to enjoy today?

WHOLE-SELF CHECKLIST
- EXERCISE
- MEAL PLAN
- ALONE TIME
- SPIRITUAL INPUT
- SCHEDULED TIME TO PROCESS AN EXPERIENCE/FEELING

TOPIC	FORMAT	SOURCE

FAVORITE FACT:

I DON'T NEED TO HAVE **ALL THE ANSWERS** TO JOIN THE **CONVERSATION**

TODAY'S DATE

TODAY'S GOAL

TODAY'S EXPLORATIONS	GIVES ENERGY	NEUTRAL	TAKES ENERGY	**T A S K S**

MUST DO THIS WEEK

What is one step I can take to better my health?

Have I put up any walls? Is there anyone I need to forgive?

What luxury can I give myself permission to enjoy today?

WHOLE-SELF CHECKLIST
- EXERCISE
- MEAL PLAN
- ALONE TIME
- SPIRITUAL INPUT
- SCHEDULED TIME TO PROCESS AN EXPERIENCE/FEELING

TOPIC	FORMAT	SOURCE

FAVORITE FACT:

I DON'T NEED TO HAVE **ALL THE ANSWERS** TO JOIN THE **CONVERSATION**

TODAY'S DATE　　　　　　　　　　**TODAY'S** GOAL

TODAY'S EXPLORATIONS	GIVES ENERGY	NEUTRAL	TAKES ENERGY	T	A	S	K	S

MUST DO THIS WEEK

What is one step I can take to better my health?

Have I put up any walls? Is there anyone I need to forgive?

What luxury can I give myself permission to enjoy today?

WHOLE-SELF CHECKLIST
- EXERCISE
- MEAL PLAN
- ALONE TIME
- SPIRITUAL INPUT
- SCHEDULED TIME TO PROCESS AN EXPERIENCE/FEELING

TOPIC	FORMAT	SOURCE

FAVORITE FACT:

I DON'T NEED TO HAVE **ALL THE ANSWERS** TO JOIN THE **CONVERSATION**

TODAY'S DATE　　　　　　　　　　　**TODAY'S** GOAL

TODAY'S EXPLORATIONS	GIVES ENERGY	NEUTRAL	TAKES ENERGY	**T A S K S**

MUST DO THIS WEEK

What is one step I can take to better my health?

Have I put up any walls? Is there anyone I need to forgive?

What luxury can I give myself permission to enjoy today?

WHOLE-SELF CHECKLIST
- EXERCISE
- MEAL PLAN
- ALONE TIME
- SPIRITUAL INPUT
- SCHEDULED TIME TO PROCESS AN EXPERIENCE/FEELING

TOPIC	FORMAT	SOURCE

FAVORITE FACT:

I DON'T NEED TO HAVE **ALL THE ANSWERS** TO JOIN THE **CONVERSATION**

TODAY'S DATE   **TODAY'S** GOAL

TODAY'S EXPLORATIONS	GIVES ENERGY	NEUTRAL	TAKES ENERGY	**T A S K S**

MUST DO THIS WEEK

What is one step I can take to better my health?

Have I put up any walls? Is there anyone I need to forgive?

What luxury can I give myself permission to enjoy today?

WHOLE-SELF CHECKLIST
- EXERCISE
- MEAL PLAN
- ALONE TIME
- SPIRITUAL INPUT
- SCHEDULED TIME TO PROCESS AN EXPERIENCE/FEELING

TOPIC	FORMAT	SOURCE

FAVORITE FACT:

I DON'T NEED TO HAVE **ALL THE ANSWERS** TO JOIN THE **CONVERSATION**

TODAY'S DATE   **TODAY'S** GOAL

TODAY'S EXPLORATIONS	GIVES ENERGY	NEUTRAL	TAKES ENERGY	**T A S K S**

MUST DO THIS WEEK

What is one step I can take to better my health?

Have I put up any walls? Is there anyone I need to forgive?

What luxury can I give myself permission to enjoy today?

WHOLE-SELF CHECKLIST
- EXERCISE
- MEAL PLAN
- ALONE TIME
- SPIRITUAL INPUT
- SCHEDULED TIME TO PROCESS AN EXPERIENCE/FEELING

TOPIC	FORMAT	SOURCE

FAVORITE FACT:

I DON'T NEED TO HAVE **ALL THE ANSWERS** TO JOIN THE **CONVERSATION**

TODAY'S DATE

TODAY'S GOAL

TODAY'S EXPLORATIONS	GIVES ENERGY	NEUTRAL	TAKES ENERGY	T A S K S

MUST DO THIS WEEK

What is one step I can take to better my health?

Have I put up any walls? Is there anyone I need to forgive?

What luxury can I give myself permission to enjoy today?

WHOLE-SELF CHECKLIST
- EXERCISE
- MEAL PLAN
- ALONE TIME
- SPIRITUAL INPUT
- SCHEDULED TIME TO PROCESS AN EXPERIENCE/FEELING

TOPIC	FORMAT	SOURCE

FAVORITE FACT:

I DON'T NEED TO HAVE **ALL THE ANSWERS** TO JOIN THE **CONVERSATION**

TODAY'S DATE

TODAY'S GOAL

TODAY'S EXPLORATIONS	GIVES ENERGY	NEUTRAL	TAKES ENERGY	T A S K S	

MUST DO THIS WEEK

What is one step I can take to better my health?

Have I put up any walls? Is there anyone I need to forgive?

What luxury can I give myself permission to enjoy today?

WHOLE-SELF CHECKLIST
- EXERCISE
- MEAL PLAN
- ALONE TIME
- SPIRITUAL INPUT
- SCHEDULED TIME TO PROCESS AN EXPERIENCE/FEELING

TOPIC	FORMAT	SOURCE

FAVORITE FACT:

I DON'T NEED TO HAVE **ALL THE ANSWERS** TO JOIN THE **CONVERSATION**

TODAY'S DATE

TODAY'S GOAL

TODAY'S EXPLORATIONS	GIVES ENERGY	NEUTRAL	TAKES ENERGY	**T** **A** **S** **K** **S**

MUST DO THIS WEEK

What is one step I can take to better my health?

Have I put up any walls? Is there anyone I need to forgive?

What luxury can I give myself permission to enjoy today?

WHOLE-SELF
C H E C K L I S T
- EXERCISE
- MEAL PLAN
- ALONE TIME
- SPIRITUAL INPUT
- SCHEDULED TIME TO PROCESS AN EXPERIENCE/FEELING

TOPIC	FORMAT	SOURCE

FAVORITE FACT:

I DON'T NEED TO HAVE **ALL THE ANSWERS** TO JOIN THE **CONVERSATION**

TODAY'S DATE | **TODAY'S** GOAL

TODAY'S EXPLORATIONS	GIVES ENERGY	NEUTRAL	TAKES ENERGY	**T A S K S**

MUST DO THIS WEEK

What is one step I can take to better my health?

Have I put up any walls? Is there anyone I need to forgive?

What luxury can I give myself permission to enjoy today?

WHOLE-SELF CHECKLIST
- EXERCISE
- MEAL PLAN
- ALONE TIME
- SPIRITUAL INPUT
- SCHEDULED TIME TO PROCESS AN EXPERIENCE/FEELING

TOPIC	FORMAT	SOURCE

FAVORITE FACT:

I DON'T NEED TO HAVE **ALL THE ANSWERS** TO JOIN THE **CONVERSATION**

TODAY'S DATE

TODAY'S GOAL

TODAY'S EXPLORATIONS	GIVES ENERGY	NEUTRAL	TAKES ENERGY

T	A	S	K	S

MUST DO THIS WEEK

What is one step I can take to better my health?

Have I put up any walls? Is there anyone I need to forgive?

What luxury can I give myself permission to enjoy today?

WHOLE-SELF CHECKLIST
- EXERCISE
- MEAL PLAN
- ALONE TIME
- SPIRITUAL INPUT
- SCHEDULED TIME TO PROCESS AN EXPERIENCE/FEELING

TOPIC	FORMAT	SOURCE

FAVORITE FACT:

I DON'T NEED TO HAVE **ALL THE ANSWERS** TO JOIN THE **CONVERSATION**

TODAY'S DATE | **TODAY'S** GOAL

TODAY'S EXPLORATIONS	GIVES ENERGY	NEUTRAL	TAKES ENERGY

T	A	S	K	S

MUST DO THIS WEEK

What is one step I can take to better my health?

Have I put up any walls? Is there anyone I need to forgive?

What luxury can I give myself permission to enjoy today?

WHOLE-SELF CHECKLIST
- EXERCISE
- MEAL PLAN
- ALONE TIME
- SPIRITUAL INPUT
- SCHEDULED TIME TO PROCESS AN EXPERIENCE/FEELING

TOPIC	FORMAT	SOURCE

FAVORITE FACT:

I DON'T NEED TO HAVE **ALL THE ANSWERS** TO JOIN THE **CONVERSATION**

TODAY'S DATE

TODAY'S GOAL

TODAY'S EXPLORATIONS	GIVES ENERGY	NEUTRAL	TAKES ENERGY

T	A	S	K	S

MUST DO THIS WEEK

What is one step I can take to better my health?

Have I put up any walls? Is there anyone I need to forgive?

What luxury can I give myself permission to enjoy today?

WHOLE-SELF CHECKLIST
- EXERCISE
- MEAL PLAN
- ALONE TIME
- SPIRITUAL INPUT
- SCHEDULED TIME TO PROCESS AN EXPERIENCE/FEELING

TOPIC	FORMAT	SOURCE

FAVORITE FACT:

I DON'T NEED TO HAVE **ALL THE ANSWERS** TO JOIN THE **CONVERSATION**

TODAY'S DATE **TODAY'S** GOAL

TODAY'S EXPLORATIONS	GIVES ENERGY	NEUTRAL	TAKES ENERGY

T	A	S	K	S

MUST DO THIS WEEK

What is one step I can take to better my health?

Have I put up any walls? Is there anyone I need to forgive?

What luxury can I give myself permission to enjoy today?

WHOLE-SELF CHECKLIST
- EXERCISE
- MEAL PLAN
- ALONE TIME
- SPIRITUAL INPUT
- SCHEDULED TIME TO PROCESS AN EXPERIENCE/FEELING

TOPIC	FORMAT	SOURCE

FAVORITE FACT:

I DON'T NEED TO HAVE **ALL THE ANSWERS** TO JOIN THE **CONVERSATION**

TODAY'S DATE

TODAY'S GOAL

TODAY'S EXPLORATIONS	GIVES ENERGY	NEUTRAL	TAKES ENERGY

T A S K S

MUST DO THIS WEEK

What is one step I can take to better my health?

Have I put up any walls? Is there anyone I need to forgive?

What luxury can I give myself permission to enjoy today?

WHOLE-SELF CHECKLIST
- EXERCISE
- MEAL PLAN
- ALONE TIME
- SPIRITUAL INPUT
- SCHEDULED TIME TO PROCESS AN EXPERIENCE/FEELING

TOPIC	FORMAT	SOURCE

FAVORITE FACT:

I DON'T NEED TO HAVE **ALL THE ANSWERS** TO JOIN THE **CONVERSATION**

TODAY'S DATE

TODAY'S GOAL

TODAY'S EXPLORATIONS	GIVES ENERGY	NEUTRAL	TAKES ENERGY	T A S K S	

MUST DO THIS WEEK

What is one step I can take to better my health?

Have I put up any walls? Is there anyone I need to forgive?

What luxury can I give myself permission to enjoy today?

WHOLE-SELF CHECKLIST
- EXERCISE
- MEAL PLAN
- ALONE TIME
- SPIRITUAL INPUT
- SCHEDULED TIME TO PROCESS AN EXPERIENCE/FEELING

TOPIC	FORMAT	SOURCE

FAVORITE FACT:

I DON'T NEED TO HAVE **ALL THE ANSWERS** TO JOIN THE **CONVERSATION**

TODAY'S DATE

TODAY'S GOAL

TODAY'S EXPLORATIONS	GIVES ENERGY	NEUTRAL	TAKES ENERGY

T A S K S

MUST DO THIS WEEK

What is one step I can take to better my health?

Have I put up any walls? Is there anyone I need to forgive?

What luxury can I give myself permission to enjoy today?

WHOLE-SELF CHECKLIST
- EXERCISE
- MEAL PLAN
- ALONE TIME
- SPIRITUAL INPUT
- SCHEDULED TIME TO PROCESS AN EXPERIENCE/FEELING

TOPIC	FORMAT	SOURCE

FAVORITE FACT:

I DON'T NEED TO HAVE **ALL THE ANSWERS** TO JOIN THE **CONVERSATION**

TODAY'S DATE | **TODAY'S** GOAL

TODAY'S EXPLORATIONS	GIVES ENERGY	NEUTRAL	TAKES ENERGY

TASKS

MUST DO THIS WEEK

What is one step I can take to better my health?

Have I put up any walls? Is there anyone I need to forgive?

What luxury can I give myself permission to enjoy today?

WHOLE-SELF CHECKLIST
- EXERCISE
- MEAL PLAN
- ALONE TIME
- SPIRITUAL INPUT
- SCHEDULED TIME TO PROCESS AN EXPERIENCE/FEELING

TOPIC	FORMAT	SOURCE

FAVORITE FACT:

I DON'T NEED TO HAVE **ALL THE ANSWERS** TO JOIN THE **CONVERSATION**

TODAY'S DATE **TODAY'S** GOAL

TODAY'S EXPLORATIONS	GIVES ENERGY	NEUTRAL	TAKES ENERGY

T A S K S

MUST DO THIS WEEK

What is one step I can take to better my health?

Have I put up any walls? Is there anyone I need to forgive?

What luxury can I give myself permission to enjoy today?

WHOLE-SELF CHECKLIST
- EXERCISE
- MEAL PLAN
- ALONE TIME
- SPIRITUAL INPUT
- SCHEDULED TIME TO PROCESS AN EXPERIENCE/FEELING

TOPIC	FORMAT	SOURCE

FAVORITE FACT:

I DON'T NEED TO HAVE **ALL THE ANSWERS** TO JOIN THE **CONVERSATION**

TODAY'S DATE

TODAY'S GOAL

TODAY'S EXPLORATIONS	GIVES ENERGY	NEUTRAL	TAKES ENERGY

T A S K S

MUST DO THIS WEEK

What is one step I can take to better my health?

Have I put up any walls? Is there anyone I need to forgive?

What luxury can I give myself permission to enjoy today?

WHOLE-SELF CHECKLIST
- EXERCISE
- MEAL PLAN
- ALONE TIME
- SPIRITUAL INPUT
- SCHEDULED TIME TO PROCESS AN EXPERIENCE/FEELING

TOPIC	FORMAT	SOURCE

FAVORITE FACT:

I DON'T NEED TO HAVE **ALL THE ANSWERS** TO JOIN THE **CONVERSATION**

TODAY'S DATE

TODAY'S GOAL

TODAY'S EXPLORATIONS	GIVES ENERGY	NEUTRAL	TAKES ENERGY	T A S K S

MUST DO THIS WEEK

What is one step I can take to better my health?

Have I put up any walls? Is there anyone I need to forgive?

What luxury can I give myself permission to enjoy today?

WHOLE-SELF CHECKLIST
- EXERCISE
- MEAL PLAN
- ALONE TIME
- SPIRITUAL INPUT
- SCHEDULED TIME TO PROCESS AN EXPERIENCE/FEELING

TOPIC	FORMAT	SOURCE

FAVORITE FACT:

I DON'T NEED TO HAVE **ALL THE ANSWERS** TO JOIN THE **CONVERSATION**

TODAY'S DATE

TODAY'S GOAL

TODAY'S EXPLORATIONS	GIVES ENERGY	NEUTRAL	TAKES ENERGY	**T A S K S**

MUST DO THIS WEEK

What is one step I can take to better my health?

Have I put up any walls? Is there anyone I need to forgive?

What luxury can I give myself permission to enjoy today?

WHOLE-SELF CHECKLIST
- EXERCISE
- MEAL PLAN
- ALONE TIME
- SPIRITUAL INPUT
- SCHEDULED TIME TO PROCESS AN EXPERIENCE/FEELING

TOPIC	FORMAT	SOURCE

FAVORITE FACT:

I DON'T NEED TO HAVE **ALL THE ANSWERS** TO JOIN THE **CONVERSATION**

TODAY'S DATE   **TODAY'S** GOAL

TODAY'S EXPLORATIONS	GIVES ENERGY	NEUTRAL	TAKES ENERGY	**T A S K S**

MUST DO THIS WEEK

What is one step I can take to better my health?

Have I put up any walls? Is there anyone I need to forgive?

What luxury can I give myself permission to enjoy today?

WHOLE-SELF CHECKLIST
- EXERCISE
- MEAL PLAN
- ALONE TIME
- SPIRITUAL INPUT
- SCHEDULED TIME TO PROCESS AN EXPERIENCE/FEELING

TOPIC	FORMAT	SOURCE

FAVORITE FACT:

I DON'T NEED TO HAVE **ALL THE ANSWERS** TO JOIN THE **CONVERSATION**

TODAY'S DATE | **TODAY'S** GOAL

TODAY'S EXPLORATIONS	GIVES ENERGY	NEUTRAL	TAKES ENERGY	T A S K S

MUST DO THIS WEEK

What is one step I can take to better my health?

Have I put up any walls? Is there anyone I need to forgive?

What luxury can I give myself permission to enjoy today?

WHOLE-SELF CHECKLIST
- EXERCISE
- MEAL PLAN
- ALONE TIME
- SPIRITUAL INPUT
- SCHEDULED TIME TO PROCESS AN EXPERIENCE/FEELING

TOPIC | FORMAT | SOURCE

FAVORITE FACT:

I DON'T NEED TO HAVE **ALL THE ANSWERS** TO JOIN THE **CONVERSATION**

TODAY'S DATE

TODAY'S GOAL

TODAY'S EXPLORATIONS	GIVES ENERGY	NEUTRAL	TAKES ENERGY

T A S K S

MUST DO THIS WEEK

What is one step I can take to better my health?

Have I put up any walls? Is there anyone I need to forgive?

What luxury can I give myself permission to enjoy today?

WHOLE-SELF CHECKLIST
- EXERCISE
- MEAL PLAN
- ALONE TIME
- SPIRITUAL INPUT
- SCHEDULED TIME TO PROCESS AN EXPERIENCE/FEELING

TOPIC	FORMAT	SOURCE

FAVORITE FACT:

I DON'T NEED TO HAVE **ALL THE ANSWERS** TO JOIN THE **CONVERSATION**

TODAY'S DATE **TODAY'S** GOAL

TODAY'S EXPLORATIONS	GIVES ENERGY	NEUTRAL	TAKES ENERGY	**T A S K S**

MUST DO THIS WEEK

What is one step I can take to better my health?

Have I put up any walls? Is there anyone I need to forgive?

What luxury can I give myself permission to enjoy today?

WHOLE-SELF CHECKLIST
- EXERCISE
- MEAL PLAN
- ALONE TIME
- SPIRITUAL INPUT
- SCHEDULED TIME TO PROCESS AN EXPERIENCE/FEELING

TOPIC	FORMAT	SOURCE

FAVORITE FACT:

I DON'T NEED TO HAVE **ALL THE ANSWERS** TO JOIN THE **CONVERSATION**

TODAY'S DATE

TODAY'S GOAL

TODAY'S EXPLORATIONS	GIVES ENERGY	NEUTRAL	TAKES ENERGY	T	A	S	K	S

MUST DO THIS WEEK

What is one step I can take to better my health?

Have I put up any walls? Is there anyone I need to forgive?

What luxury can I give myself permission to enjoy today?

WHOLE-SELF CHECKLIST
- EXERCISE
- MEAL PLAN
- ALONE TIME
- SPIRITUAL INPUT
- SCHEDULED TIME TO PROCESS AN EXPERIENCE/FEELING

TOPIC	FORMAT	SOURCE

FAVORITE FACT:

I DON'T NEED TO HAVE **ALL THE ANSWERS** TO JOIN THE **CONVERSATION**

TODAY'S DATE | **TODAY'S** GOAL

TODAY'S EXPLORATIONS	GIVES ENERGY	NEUTRAL	TAKES ENERGY	T A S K S	

MUST DO THIS WEEK

What is one step I can take to better my health?

Have I put up any walls? Is there anyone I need to forgive?

What luxury can I give myself permission to enjoy today?

WHOLE-SELF CHECKLIST
- EXERCISE
- MEAL PLAN
- ALONE TIME
- SPIRITUAL INPUT
- SCHEDULED TIME TO PROCESS AN EXPERIENCE/FEELING

TOPIC	FORMAT	SOURCE

FAVORITE FACT:

I DON'T NEED TO HAVE **ALL THE ANSWERS** TO JOIN THE **CONVERSATION**

TODAY'S DATE **TODAY'S** GOAL

TODAY'S EXPLORATIONS	GIVES ENERGY	NEUTRAL	TAKES ENERGY	T A S K S

MUST DO THIS WEEK

What is one step I can take to better my health?

Have I put up any walls? Is there anyone I need to forgive?

What luxury can I give myself permission to enjoy today?

WHOLE-SELF CHECKLIST
- EXERCISE
- MEAL PLAN
- ALONE TIME
- SPIRITUAL INPUT
- SCHEDULED TIME TO PROCESS AN EXPERIENCE/FEELING

TOPIC	FORMAT	SOURCE

FAVORITE FACT:

I DON'T NEED TO HAVE **ALL THE ANSWERS** TO JOIN THE **CONVERSATION**

TODAY'S DATE | **TODAY'S** GOAL

TODAY'S EXPLORATIONS	GIVES ENERGY	NEUTRAL	TAKES ENERGY	**T A S K S**

MUST DO THIS WEEK

What is one step I can take to better my health?

Have I put up any walls? Is there anyone I need to forgive?

What luxury can I give myself permission to enjoy today?

WHOLE-SELF CHECKLIST
- EXERCISE
- MEAL PLAN
- ALONE TIME
- SPIRITUAL INPUT
- SCHEDULED TIME TO PROCESS AN EXPERIENCE/FEELING

TOPIC	FORMAT	SOURCE

FAVORITE FACT:

I DON'T NEED TO HAVE **ALL THE ANSWERS** TO JOIN THE **CONVERSATION**

TODAY'S DATE

TODAY'S GOAL

TODAY'S EXPLORATIONS	GIVES ENERGY	NEUTRAL	TAKES ENERGY

TASKS

MUST DO THIS WEEK

What is one step I can take to better my health?

Have I put up any walls? Is there anyone I need to forgive?

What luxury can I give myself permission to enjoy today?

WHOLE-SELF CHECKLIST
- EXERCISE
- MEAL PLAN
- ALONE TIME
- SPIRITUAL INPUT
- SCHEDULED TIME TO PROCESS AN EXPERIENCE/FEELING

TOPIC	FORMAT	SOURCE

FAVORITE FACT:

I DON'T NEED TO HAVE **ALL THE ANSWERS** TO JOIN THE **CONVERSATION**

TODAY'S DATE

TODAY'S GOAL

TODAY'S EXPLORATIONS	GIVES ENERGY	NEUTRAL	TAKES ENERGY

TASKS

MUST DO THIS WEEK

What is one step I can take to better my health?

Have I put up any walls? Is there anyone I need to forgive?

What luxury can I give myself permission to enjoy today?

WHOLE-SELF CHECKLIST
- EXERCISE
- MEAL PLAN
- ALONE TIME
- SPIRITUAL INPUT
- SCHEDULED TIME TO PROCESS AN EXPERIENCE/FEELING

TOPIC	FORMAT	SOURCE

FAVORITE FACT:

I DON'T NEED TO HAVE **ALL THE ANSWERS** TO JOIN THE **CONVERSATION**

TODAY'S DATE

TODAY'S GOAL

TODAY'S EXPLORATIONS	GIVES ENERGY	NEUTRAL	TAKES ENERGY	**T A S K S**

MUST DO THIS WEEK

What is one step I can take to better my health?

Have I put up any walls? Is there anyone I need to forgive?

What luxury can I give myself permission to enjoy today?

WHOLE-SELF CHECKLIST
- EXERCISE
- MEAL PLAN
- ALONE TIME
- SPIRITUAL INPUT
- SCHEDULED TIME TO PROCESS AN EXPERIENCE/FEELING

TOPIC	FORMAT	SOURCE

FAVORITE FACT:

I DON'T NEED TO HAVE **ALL THE ANSWERS** TO JOIN THE **CONVERSATION**

TODAY'S DATE   **TODAY'S** GOAL

TODAY'S EXPLORATIONS	GIVES ENERGY	NEUTRAL	TAKES ENERGY	**T A S K S**

MUST DO THIS WEEK

What is one step I can take to better my health?

Have I put up any walls? Is there anyone I need to forgive?

What luxury can I give myself permission to enjoy today?

WHOLE-SELF CHECKLIST
- EXERCISE
- MEAL PLAN
- ALONE TIME
- SPIRITUAL INPUT
- SCHEDULED TIME TO PROCESS AN EXPERIENCE/FEELING

TOPIC   FORMAT   SOURCE

FAVORITE FACT:

I DON'T NEED TO HAVE **ALL THE ANSWERS** TO JOIN THE **CONVERSATION**

TODAY'S DATE

TODAY'S GOAL

TODAY'S EXPLORATIONS	GIVES ENERGY	NEUTRAL	TAKES ENERGY

T A S K S

MUST DO THIS WEEK

What is one step I can take to better my health?

Have I put up any walls? Is there anyone I need to forgive?

What luxury can I give myself permission to enjoy today?

WHOLE-SELF CHECKLIST
- EXERCISE
- MEAL PLAN
- ALONE TIME
- SPIRITUAL INPUT
- SCHEDULED TIME TO PROCESS AN EXPERIENCE/FEELING

TOPIC	FORMAT	SOURCE

FAVORITE FACT:

I DON'T NEED TO HAVE **ALL THE ANSWERS** TO JOIN THE **CONVERSATION**

TODAY'S DATE   **TODAY'S** GOAL

TODAY'S EXPLORATIONS	GIVES ENERGY	NEUTRAL	TAKES ENERGY	T A S K S	

MUST DO THIS WEEK

What is one step I can take to better my health?

WHOLE-SELF CHECKLIST

Have I put up any walls? Is there anyone I need to forgive?

- EXERCISE
- MEAL PLAN
- ALONE TIME

What luxury can I give myself permission to enjoy today?

- SPIRITUAL INPUT
- SCHEDULED TIME TO PROCESS AN EXPERIENCE/FEELING

TOPIC	FORMAT	SOURCE

FAVORITE FACT:

I DON'T NEED TO HAVE **ALL THE ANSWERS** TO JOIN THE **CONVERSATION**

TODAY'S DATE

TODAY'S GOAL

TODAY'S EXPLORATIONS	GIVES ENERGY	NEUTRAL	TAKES ENERGY	**T A S K S**

MUST DO THIS WEEK

What is one step I can take to better my health?

Have I put up any walls? Is there anyone I need to forgive?

What luxury can I give myself permission to enjoy today?

WHOLE-SELF
C H E C K L I S T
- EXERCISE
- MEAL PLAN
- ALONE TIME
- SPIRITUAL INPUT
- SCHEDULED TIME TO PROCESS AN EXPERIENCE/FEELING

TOPIC	FORMAT	SOURCE

FAVORITE FACT:

I DON'T NEED TO HAVE **ALL THE ANSWERS** TO JOIN THE **CONVERSATION**

TODAY'S DATE   **TODAY'S** GOAL

TODAY'S EXPLORATIONS	GIVES ENERGY	NEUTRAL	TAKES ENERGY

TASKS

MUST DO THIS WEEK

What is one step I can take to better my health?

Have I put up any walls? Is there anyone I need to forgive?

What luxury can I give myself permission to enjoy today?

WHOLE-SELF CHECKLIST
- EXERCISE
- MEAL PLAN
- ALONE TIME
- SPIRITUAL INPUT
- SCHEDULED TIME TO PROCESS AN EXPERIENCE/FEELING

TOPIC	FORMAT	SOURCE

FAVORITE FACT:

I DON'T NEED TO HAVE **ALL THE ANSWERS** TO JOIN THE **CONVERSATION**

TODAY'S DATE   **TODAY'S** GOAL

TODAY'S EXPLORATIONS	GIVES ENERGY	NEUTRAL	TAKES ENERGY	TASKS

MUST DO THIS WEEK

What is one step I can take to better my health?

Have I put up any walls? Is there anyone I need to forgive?

What luxury can I give myself permission to enjoy today?

WHOLE-SELF CHECKLIST
- EXERCISE
- MEAL PLAN
- ALONE TIME
- SPIRITUAL INPUT
- SCHEDULED TIME TO PROCESS AN EXPERIENCE/FEELING

TOPIC	FORMAT	SOURCE

FAVORITE FACT:

I DON'T NEED TO HAVE **ALL THE ANSWERS** TO JOIN THE **CONVERSATION**

TODAY'S DATE

TODAY'S GOAL

TODAY'S EXPLORATIONS	GIVES ENERGY	NEUTRAL	TAKES ENERGY

T A S K S

MUST DO THIS WEEK

What is one step I can take to better my health?

Have I put up any walls? Is there anyone I need to forgive?

What luxury can I give myself permission to enjoy today?

WHOLE-SELF
C H E C K L I S T
- EXERCISE
- MEAL PLAN
- ALONE TIME
- SPIRITUAL INPUT
- SCHEDULED TIME TO PROCESS AN EXPERIENCE/FEELING

TOPIC	FORMAT	SOURCE

FAVORITE FACT:

I DON'T NEED TO HAVE **ALL THE ANSWERS** TO JOIN THE **CONVERSATION**

TODAY'S DATE

TODAY'S GOAL

TODAY'S EXPLORATIONS	GIVES ENERGY	NEUTRAL	TAKES ENERGY	**T A S K S**

MUST DO THIS WEEK

What is one step I can take to better my health?

Have I put up any walls? Is there anyone I need to forgive?

What luxury can I give myself permission to enjoy today?

WHOLE-SELF CHECKLIST
- EXERCISE
- MEAL PLAN
- ALONE TIME
- SPIRITUAL INPUT
- SCHEDULED TIME TO PROCESS AN EXPERIENCE/FEELING

TOPIC	FORMAT	SOURCE

FAVORITE FACT:

I DON'T NEED TO HAVE **ALL THE ANSWERS** TO JOIN THE **CONVERSATION**

TODAY'S DATE

TODAY'S GOAL

TODAY'S EXPLORATIONS	GIVES ENERGY	NEUTRAL	TAKES ENERGY	**T A S K S**

MUST DO THIS WEEK

What is one step I can take to better my health?

Have I put up any walls? Is there anyone I need to forgive?

What luxury can I give myself permission to enjoy today?

WHOLE-SELF CHECKLIST
- EXERCISE
- MEAL PLAN
- ALONE TIME
- SPIRITUAL INPUT
- SCHEDULED TIME TO PROCESS AN EXPERIENCE/FEELING

TOPIC	FORMAT	SOURCE

FAVORITE FACT:

I DON'T NEED TO HAVE **ALL THE ANSWERS** TO JOIN THE **CONVERSATION**

TODAY'S DATE | **TODAY'S** GOAL

TODAY'S EXPLORATIONS	GIVES ENERGY	NEUTRAL	TAKES ENERGY	**T A S K S**

MUST DO THIS WEEK

What is one step I can take to better my health?

Have I put up any walls? Is there anyone I need to forgive?

What luxury can I give myself permission to enjoy today?

WHOLE-SELF CHECKLIST
- EXERCISE
- MEAL PLAN
- ALONE TIME
- SPIRITUAL INPUT
- SCHEDULED TIME TO PROCESS AN EXPERIENCE/FEELING

TOPIC	FORMAT	SOURCE

FAVORITE FACT:

I DON'T NEED TO HAVE **ALL THE ANSWERS** TO JOIN THE **CONVERSATION**

TODAY'S DATE

TODAY'S GOAL

TODAY'S EXPLORATIONS	GIVES ENERGY	NEUTRAL	TAKES ENERGY

T A S K S

MUST DO THIS WEEK

What is one step I can take to better my health?

Have I put up any walls? Is there anyone I need to forgive?

What luxury can I give myself permission to enjoy today?

WHOLE-SELF CHECKLIST
- EXERCISE
- MEAL PLAN
- ALONE TIME
- SPIRITUAL INPUT
- SCHEDULED TIME TO PROCESS AN EXPERIENCE/FEELING

TOPIC	FORMAT	SOURCE

FAVORITE FACT:

I DON'T NEED TO HAVE **ALL THE ANSWERS** TO JOIN THE **CONVERSATION**

TODAY'S DATE

TODAY'S GOAL

TODAY'S EXPLORATIONS	GIVES ENERGY	NEUTRAL	TAKES ENERGY

T A S K S

MUST DO THIS WEEK

What is one step I can take to better my health?

Have I put up any walls? Is there anyone I need to forgive?

What luxury can I give myself permission to enjoy today?

WHOLE-SELF CHECKLIST
- EXERCISE
- MEAL PLAN
- ALONE TIME
- SPIRITUAL INPUT
- SCHEDULED TIME TO PROCESS AN EXPERIENCE/FEELING

TOPIC	FORMAT	SOURCE

FAVORITE FACT:

I DON'T NEED TO HAVE **ALL THE ANSWERS** TO JOIN THE **CONVERSATION**

TODAY'S DATE | **TODAY'S** GOAL

TODAY'S EXPLORATIONS	GIVES ENERGY	NEUTRAL	TAKES ENERGY	**T A S K S**

MUST DO THIS WEEK

What is one step I can take to better my health?

Have I put up any walls? Is there anyone I need to forgive?

What luxury can I give myself permission to enjoy today?

WHOLE-SELF CHECKLIST
- EXERCISE
- MEAL PLAN
- ALONE TIME
- SPIRITUAL INPUT
- SCHEDULED TIME TO PROCESS AN EXPERIENCE/FEELING

TOPIC	FORMAT	SOURCE

FAVORITE FACT:

I DON'T NEED TO HAVE **ALL THE ANSWERS** TO JOIN THE **CONVERSATION**

TODAY'S DATE

TODAY'S GOAL

TODAY'S EXPLORATIONS	GIVES ENERGY	NEUTRAL	TAKES ENERGY	**T A S K S**

MUST DO THIS WEEK

What is one step I can take to better my health?

Have I put up any walls? Is there anyone I need to forgive?

What luxury can I give myself permission to enjoy today?

WHOLE-SELF CHECKLIST
- EXERCISE
- MEAL PLAN
- ALONE TIME
- SPIRITUAL INPUT
- SCHEDULED TIME TO PROCESS AN EXPERIENCE/FEELING

TOPIC	FORMAT	SOURCE

FAVORITE FACT:

I DON'T NEED TO HAVE **ALL THE ANSWERS** TO JOIN THE **CONVERSATION**

TODAY'S DATE | **TODAY'S** GOAL

TODAY'S EXPLORATIONS	GIVES ENERGY	NEUTRAL	TAKES ENERGY

TASKS

MUST DO THIS WEEK

What is one step I can take to better my health?

Have I put up any walls? Is there anyone I need to forgive?

What luxury can I give myself permission to enjoy today?

WHOLE-SELF CHECKLIST
- EXERCISE
- MEAL PLAN
- ALONE TIME
- SPIRITUAL INPUT
- SCHEDULED TIME TO PROCESS AN EXPERIENCE/FEELING

TOPIC	FORMAT	SOURCE

FAVORITE FACT:

I DON'T NEED TO HAVE **ALL THE ANSWERS** TO JOIN THE **CONVERSATION**

TODAY'S DATE

TODAY'S GOAL

TODAY'S EXPLORATIONS	GIVES ENERGY	NEUTRAL	TAKES ENERGY

T A S K S

MUST DO THIS WEEK

What is one step I can take to better my health?

Have I put up any walls? Is there anyone I need to forgive?

What luxury can I give myself permission to enjoy today?

WHOLE-SELF
C H E C K L I S T
- EXERCISE
- MEAL PLAN
- ALONE TIME
- SPIRITUAL INPUT
- SCHEDULED TIME TO PROCESS AN EXPERIENCE/FEELING

TOPIC

FORMAT

SOURCE

FAVORITE FACT:

I DON'T NEED TO HAVE **ALL THE ANSWERS** TO JOIN THE **CONVERSATION**

TODAY'S DATE

TODAY'S GOAL

TODAY'S EXPLORATIONS	GIVES ENERGY	NEUTRAL	TAKES ENERGY	**T A S K S**

MUST DO THIS WEEK

What is one step I can take to better my health?

Have I put up any walls? Is there anyone I need to forgive?

What luxury can I give myself permission to enjoy today?

WHOLE-SELF CHECKLIST
- EXERCISE
- MEAL PLAN
- ALONE TIME
- SPIRITUAL INPUT
- SCHEDULED TIME TO PROCESS AN EXPERIENCE/FEELING

TOPIC	FORMAT	SOURCE

FAVORITE FACT:

I DON'T NEED TO HAVE **ALL THE ANSWERS** TO JOIN THE **CONVERSATION**

TODAY'S DATE

TODAY'S GOAL

TODAY'S EXPLORATIONS	GIVES ENERGY	NEUTRAL	TAKES ENERGY

T A S K S

MUST DO THIS WEEK

What is one step I can take to better my health?

Have I put up any walls? Is there anyone I need to forgive?

What luxury can I give myself permission to enjoy today?

WHOLE-SELF CHECKLIST
- EXERCISE
- MEAL PLAN
- ALONE TIME
- SPIRITUAL INPUT
- SCHEDULED TIME TO PROCESS AN EXPERIENCE/FEELING

TOPIC	FORMAT	SOURCE

FAVORITE FACT:

I DON'T NEED TO HAVE **ALL THE ANSWERS** TO JOIN THE **CONVERSATION**

TODAY'S DATE

TODAY'S GOAL

TODAY'S EXPLORATIONS	GIVES ENERGY	NEUTRAL	TAKES ENERGY

T A S K S

MUST DO THIS WEEK

What is one step I can take to better my health?

Have I put up any walls? Is there anyone I need to forgive?

What luxury can I give myself permission to enjoy today?

WHOLE-SELF
C H E C K L I S T
- EXERCISE
- MEAL PLAN
- ALONE TIME
- SPIRITUAL INPUT
- SCHEDULED TIME TO PROCESS AN EXPERIENCE/FEELING

TOPIC	FORMAT	SOURCE

FAVORITE FACT:

I DON'T NEED TO HAVE **ALL THE ANSWERS** TO JOIN THE **CONVERSATION**

TODAY'S DATE

TODAY'S GOAL

TODAY'S EXPLORATIONS	GIVES ENERGY	NEUTRAL	TAKES ENERGY	**T A S K S**

MUST DO THIS WEEK

What is one step I can take to better my health?

Have I put up any walls? Is there anyone I need to forgive?

What luxury can I give myself permission to enjoy today?

WHOLE-SELF CHECKLIST
- EXERCISE
- MEAL PLAN
- ALONE TIME
- SPIRITUAL INPUT
- SCHEDULED TIME TO PROCESS AN EXPERIENCE/FEELING

TOPIC	FORMAT	SOURCE

FAVORITE FACT:

I DON'T NEED TO HAVE **ALL THE ANSWERS** TO JOIN THE **CONVERSATION**

TODAY'S DATE

TODAY'S GOAL

TODAY'S EXPLORATIONS	GIVES ENERGY	NEUTRAL	TAKES ENERGY

T A S K S

MUST DO THIS WEEK

What is one step I can take to better my health?

Have I put up any walls? Is there anyone I need to forgive?

What luxury can I give myself permission to enjoy today?

WHOLE-SELF CHECKLIST
- EXERCISE
- MEAL PLAN
- ALONE TIME
- SPIRITUAL INPUT
- SCHEDULED TIME TO PROCESS AN EXPERIENCE/FEELING

TOPIC	FORMAT	SOURCE

FAVORITE FACT:

I DON'T NEED TO HAVE **ALL THE ANSWERS** TO JOIN THE **CONVERSATION**

TODAY'S DATE

TODAY'S GOAL

TODAY'S EXPLORATIONS	GIVES ENERGY	NEUTRAL	TAKES ENERGY

T A S K S

MUST DO THIS WEEK

What is one step I can take to better my health?

Have I put up any walls? Is there anyone I need to forgive?

What luxury can I give myself permission to enjoy today?

WHOLE-SELF CHECKLIST
- EXERCISE
- MEAL PLAN
- ALONE TIME
- SPIRITUAL INPUT
- SCHEDULED TIME TO PROCESS AN EXPERIENCE/FEELING

TOPIC	FORMAT	SOURCE

FAVORITE FACT:

I DON'T NEED TO HAVE **ALL THE ANSWERS** TO JOIN THE **CONVERSATION**

TODAY'S DATE

TODAY'S GOAL

TODAY'S EXPLORATIONS	GIVES ENERGY	NEUTRAL	TAKES ENERGY

T	A	S	K	S

MUST DO THIS WEEK

What is one step I can take to better my health?

Have I put up any walls? Is there anyone I need to forgive?

What luxury can I give myself permission to enjoy today?

WHOLE-SELF
CHECKLIST
- EXERCISE
- MEAL PLAN
- ALONE TIME
- SPIRITUAL INPUT
- SCHEDULED TIME TO PROCESS AN EXPERIENCE/FEELING

TOPIC	FORMAT	SOURCE

FAVORITE FACT:

I DON'T NEED TO HAVE **ALL THE ANSWERS** TO JOIN THE **CONVERSATION**

TODAY'S DATE

TODAY'S GOAL

TODAY'S EXPLORATIONS	GIVES ENERGY	NEUTRAL	TAKES ENERGY	**T A S K S**

MUST DO THIS WEEK

What is one step I can take to better my health?

Have I put up any walls? Is there anyone I need to forgive?

What luxury can I give myself permission to enjoy today?

WHOLE-SELF CHECKLIST
- EXERCISE
- MEAL PLAN
- ALONE TIME
- SPIRITUAL INPUT
- SCHEDULED TIME TO PROCESS AN EXPERIENCE/FEELING

TOPIC	FORMAT	SOURCE

FAVORITE FACT:

I DON'T NEED TO HAVE **ALL THE ANSWERS** TO JOIN THE **CONVERSATION**

TODAY'S DATE

TODAY'S GOAL

TODAY'S EXPLORATIONS	GIVES ENERGY	NEUTRAL	TAKES ENERGY	**T A S K S**

MUST DO THIS WEEK

What is one step I can take to better my health?

Have I put up any walls? Is there anyone I need to forgive?

What luxury can I give myself permission to enjoy today?

WHOLE-SELF
C H E C K L I S T
- EXERCISE
- MEAL PLAN
- ALONE TIME
- SPIRITUAL INPUT
- SCHEDULED TIME TO PROCESS AN EXPERIENCE/FEELING

TOPIC	FORMAT	SOURCE

FAVORITE FACT:

I DON'T NEED TO HAVE **ALL THE ANSWERS** TO JOIN THE **CONVERSATION**

TODAY'S DATE   **TODAY'S** GOAL

TODAY'S EXPLORATIONS	GIVES ENERGY	NEUTRAL	TAKES ENERGY	T A S K S

MUST DO THIS WEEK

What is one step I can take to better my health?

Have I put up any walls? Is there anyone I need to forgive?

What luxury can I give myself permission to enjoy today?

WHOLE-SELF CHECKLIST
- EXERCISE
- MEAL PLAN
- ALONE TIME
- SPIRITUAL INPUT
- SCHEDULED TIME TO PROCESS AN EXPERIENCE/FEELING

TOPIC	FORMAT	SOURCE

FAVORITE FACT:

I DON'T NEED TO HAVE **ALL THE ANSWERS** TO JOIN THE **CONVERSATION**

TODAY'S DATE **TODAY'S** GOAL

TODAY'S EXPLORATIONS	GIVES ENERGY	NEUTRAL	TAKES ENERGY	T A S K S
				MUST DO THIS WEEK

What is one step I can take to better my health?

Have I put up any walls? Is there anyone I need to forgive?

What luxury can I give myself permission to enjoy today?

WHOLE-SELF CHECKLIST
- EXERCISE
- MEAL PLAN
- ALONE TIME
- SPIRITUAL INPUT
- SCHEDULED TIME TO PROCESS AN EXPERIENCE/FEELING

TOPIC	FORMAT	SOURCE

FAVORITE FACT:

I DON'T NEED TO HAVE **ALL THE ANSWERS** TO JOIN THE **CONVERSATION**

TODAY'S DATE

TODAY'S GOAL

TODAY'S EXPLORATIONS	GIVES ENERGY	NEUTRAL	TAKES ENERGY

T	**A**	**S**	**K**	**S**

MUST DO THIS WEEK

What is one step I can take to better my health?

Have I put up any walls? Is there anyone I need to forgive?

What luxury can I give myself permission to enjoy today?

WHOLE-SELF CHECKLIST
- EXERCISE
- MEAL PLAN
- ALONE TIME
- SPIRITUAL INPUT
- SCHEDULED TIME TO PROCESS AN EXPERIENCE/FEELING

TOPIC	FORMAT	SOURCE

FAVORITE FACT:

I DON'T NEED TO HAVE **ALL THE ANSWERS** TO JOIN THE **CONVERSATION**

TODAY'S DATE

TODAY'S GOAL

TODAY'S EXPLORATIONS	GIVES ENERGY	NEUTRAL	TAKES ENERGY

T A S K S

MUST DO THIS WEEK

What is one step I can take to better my health?

Have I put up any walls? Is there anyone I need to forgive?

What luxury can I give myself permission to enjoy today?

WHOLE-SELF
C H E C K L I S T
- EXERCISE
- MEAL PLAN
- ALONE TIME
- SPIRITUAL INPUT
- SCHEDULED TIME TO PROCESS AN EXPERIENCE/FEELING

TOPIC	FORMAT	SOURCE

FAVORITE FACT:

I DON'T NEED TO HAVE **ALL THE ANSWERS** TO JOIN THE **CONVERSATION**

TODAY'S DATE **TODAY'S** GOAL

TODAY'S EXPLORATIONS	GIVES ENERGY	NEUTRAL	TAKES ENERGY	T A S K S

MUST DO THIS WEEK

What is one step I can take to better my health?

Have I put up any walls? Is there anyone I need to forgive?

What luxury can I give myself permission to enjoy today?

WHOLE-SELF CHECKLIST
- EXERCISE
- MEAL PLAN
- ALONE TIME
- SPIRITUAL INPUT
- SCHEDULED TIME TO PROCESS AN EXPERIENCE/FEELING

TOPIC	FORMAT	SOURCE

FAVORITE FACT:

I DON'T NEED TO HAVE **ALL THE ANSWERS** TO JOIN THE **CONVERSATION**

TODAY'S DATE | **TODAY'S** GOAL

TODAY'S EXPLORATIONS	GIVES ENERGY	NEUTRAL	TAKES ENERGY

T A S K S

MUST DO THIS WEEK

What is one step I can take to better my health?

Have I put up any walls? Is there anyone I need to forgive?

What luxury can I give myself permission to enjoy today?

WHOLE-SELF CHECKLIST
- EXERCISE
- MEAL PLAN
- ALONE TIME
- SPIRITUAL INPUT
- SCHEDULED TIME TO PROCESS AN EXPERIENCE/FEELING

TOPIC	FORMAT	SOURCE

FAVORITE FACT:

I DON'T NEED TO HAVE **ALL THE ANSWERS** TO JOIN THE **CONVERSATION**

TODAY'S DATE

TODAY'S GOAL

TODAY'S EXPLORATIONS	GIVES ENERGY	NEUTRAL	TAKES ENERGY

T A S K S

MUST DO THIS WEEK

What is one step I can take to better my health?

Have I put up any walls? Is there anyone I need to forgive?

What luxury can I give myself permission to enjoy today?

WHOLE-SELF CHECKLIST
- EXERCISE
- MEAL PLAN
- ALONE TIME
- SPIRITUAL INPUT
- SCHEDULED TIME TO PROCESS AN EXPERIENCE/FEELING

TOPIC	FORMAT	SOURCE

FAVORITE FACT:

I DON'T NEED TO HAVE **ALL THE ANSWERS** TO JOIN THE **CONVERSATION**

TODAY'S DATE   **TODAY'S** GOAL

TODAY'S EXPLORATIONS	GIVES ENERGY	NEUTRAL	TAKES ENERGY	T A S K S

MUST DO THIS WEEK

What is one step I can take to better my health?

Have I put up any walls? Is there anyone I need to forgive?

What luxury can I give myself permission to enjoy today?

WHOLE-SELF CHECKLIST
- EXERCISE
- MEAL PLAN
- ALONE TIME
- SPIRITUAL INPUT
- SCHEDULED TIME TO PROCESS AN EXPERIENCE/FEELING

TOPIC	FORMAT	SOURCE

FAVORITE FACT:

I DON'T NEED TO HAVE **ALL THE ANSWERS** TO JOIN THE **CONVERSATION**

TODAY'S DATE

TODAY'S GOAL

TODAY'S EXPLORATIONS	GIVES ENERGY	NEUTRAL	TAKES ENERGY	**T**	**A**	**S**	**K**	**S**

MUST DO THIS WEEK

What is one step I can take to better my health?

Have I put up any walls? Is there anyone I need to forgive?

What luxury can I give myself permission to enjoy today?

WHOLE-SELF CHECKLIST
- EXERCISE
- MEAL PLAN
- ALONE TIME
- SPIRITUAL INPUT
- SCHEDULED TIME TO PROCESS AN EXPERIENCE/FEELING

TOPIC	FORMAT	SOURCE

FAVORITE FACT:

I DON'T NEED TO HAVE **ALL THE ANSWERS** TO JOIN THE **CONVERSATION**

TODAY'S DATE

TODAY'S GOAL

TODAY'S EXPLORATIONS	GIVES ENERGY	NEUTRAL	TAKES ENERGY	T A S K S

MUST DO THIS WEEK

What is one step I can take to better my health?

Have I put up any walls? Is there anyone I need to forgive?

What luxury can I give myself permission to enjoy today?

WHOLE-SELF CHECKLIST
- EXERCISE
- MEAL PLAN
- ALONE TIME
- SPIRITUAL INPUT
- SCHEDULED TIME TO PROCESS AN EXPERIENCE/FEELING

TOPIC	FORMAT	SOURCE

FAVORITE FACT:

I DON'T NEED TO HAVE **ALL THE ANSWERS** TO JOIN THE **CONVERSATION**

TODAY'S DATE

TODAY'S GOAL

TODAY'S EXPLORATIONS	GIVES ENERGY	NEUTRAL	TAKES ENERGY

T A S K S

MUST DO THIS WEEK

What is one step I can take to better my health?

Have I put up any walls? Is there anyone I need to forgive?

What luxury can I give myself permission to enjoy today?

WHOLE-SELF CHECKLIST
- EXERCISE
- MEAL PLAN
- ALONE TIME
- SPIRITUAL INPUT
- SCHEDULED TIME TO PROCESS AN EXPERIENCE/FEELING

TOPIC	FORMAT	SOURCE

FAVORITE FACT:

I DON'T NEED TO HAVE **ALL THE ANSWERS** TO JOIN THE **CONVERSATION**

TODAY'S DATE

TODAY'S GOAL

TODAY'S EXPLORATIONS	GIVES ENERGY	NEUTRAL	TAKES ENERGY	**T A S K S**

MUST DO THIS WEEK

What is one step I can take to better my health?

Have I put up any walls? Is there anyone I need to forgive?

What luxury can I give myself permission to enjoy today?

WHOLE-SELF CHECKLIST
- EXERCISE
- MEAL PLAN
- ALONE TIME
- SPIRITUAL INPUT
- SCHEDULED TIME TO PROCESS AN EXPERIENCE/FEELING

TOPIC	FORMAT	SOURCE

FAVORITE FACT:

I DON'T NEED TO HAVE **ALL THE ANSWERS** TO JOIN THE **CONVERSATION**

TODAY'S DATE **TODAY'S** GOAL

TODAY'S EXPLORATIONS	GIVES ENERGY	NEUTRAL	TAKES ENERGY	**T A S K S**

MUST DO THIS WEEK

What is one step I can take to better my health?

Have I put up any walls? Is there anyone I need to forgive?

What luxury can I give myself permission to enjoy today?

WHOLE-SELF CHECKLIST
- EXERCISE
- MEAL PLAN
- ALONE TIME
- SPIRITUAL INPUT
- SCHEDULED TIME TO PROCESS AN EXPERIENCE/FEELING

TOPIC	FORMAT	SOURCE

FAVORITE FACT:

I DON'T NEED TO HAVE **ALL THE ANSWERS** TO JOIN THE **CONVERSATION**

TODAY'S DATE

TODAY'S GOAL

TODAY'S EXPLORATIONS	GIVES ENERGY	NEUTRAL	TAKES ENERGY	T A S K S

MUST DO THIS WEEK

What is one step I can take to better my health?

Have I put up any walls? Is there anyone I need to forgive?

What luxury can I give myself permission to enjoy today?

WHOLE-SELF CHECKLIST
- EXERCISE
- MEAL PLAN
- ALONE TIME
- SPIRITUAL INPUT
- SCHEDULED TIME TO PROCESS AN EXPERIENCE/FEELING

TOPIC	FORMAT	SOURCE

FAVORITE FACT:

I DON'T NEED TO HAVE **ALL THE ANSWERS** TO JOIN THE **CONVERSATION**

TODAY'S DATE   **TODAY'S** GOAL

TODAY'S EXPLORATIONS	GIVES ENERGY	NEUTRAL	TAKES ENERGY	**T A S K S**

MUST DO THIS WEEK

What is one step I can take to better my health?

Have I put up any walls? Is there anyone I need to forgive?

What luxury can I give myself permission to enjoy today?

WHOLE-SELF
C H E C K L I S T
- EXERCISE
- MEAL PLAN
- ALONE TIME
- SPIRITUAL INPUT
- SCHEDULED TIME TO PROCESS AN EXPERIENCE/FEELING

TOPIC	FORMAT	SOURCE

FAVORITE FACT:

I DON'T NEED TO HAVE **ALL THE ANSWERS** TO JOIN THE **CONVERSATION**

TODAY'S DATE

TODAY'S GOAL

TODAY'S EXPLORATIONS	GIVES ENERGY	NEUTRAL	TAKES ENERGY

T A S K S

MUST DO THIS WEEK

What is one step I can take to better my health?

Have I put up any walls? Is there anyone I need to forgive?

What luxury can I give myself permission to enjoy today?

WHOLE-SELF CHECKLIST
- EXERCISE
- MEAL PLAN
- ALONE TIME
- SPIRITUAL INPUT
- SCHEDULED TIME TO PROCESS AN EXPERIENCE/FEELING

TOPIC	FORMAT	SOURCE

FAVORITE FACT:

I DON'T NEED TO HAVE **ALL THE ANSWERS** TO JOIN THE **CONVERSATION**

TODAY'S DATE **TODAY'S** GOAL

TODAY'S EXPLORATIONS	GIVES ENERGY	NEUTRAL	TAKES ENERGY	**T**	**A**	**S**	**K**	**S**

MUST DO THIS WEEK

What is one step I can take to better my health?

Have I put up any walls? Is there anyone I need to forgive?

What luxury can I give myself permission to enjoy today?

WHOLE-SELF CHECKLIST
- EXERCISE
- MEAL PLAN
- ALONE TIME
- SPIRITUAL INPUT
- SCHEDULED TIME TO PROCESS AN EXPERIENCE/FEELING

TOPIC	FORMAT	SOURCE

FAVORITE FACT:

I DON'T NEED TO HAVE **ALL THE ANSWERS** TO JOIN THE **CONVERSATION**

TODAY'S DATE | **TODAY'S** GOAL

TODAY'S EXPLORATIONS	GIVES ENERGY	NEUTRAL	TAKES ENERGY

T	A	S	K	S

MUST DO THIS WEEK

What is one step I can take to better my health?

Have I put up any walls? Is there anyone I need to forgive?

What luxury can I give myself permission to enjoy today?

WHOLE-SELF CHECKLIST
- EXERCISE
- MEAL PLAN
- ALONE TIME
- SPIRITUAL INPUT
- SCHEDULED TIME TO PROCESS AN EXPERIENCE/FEELING

TOPIC	FORMAT	SOURCE

FAVORITE FACT:

I DON'T NEED TO HAVE **ALL THE ANSWERS** TO JOIN THE **CONVERSATION**

TODAY'S DATE

TODAY'S GOAL

TODAY'S EXPLORATIONS	GIVES ENERGY	NEUTRAL	TAKES ENERGY	T A S K S

MUST DO THIS WEEK

What is one step I can take to better my health?

Have I put up any walls? Is there anyone I need to forgive?

What luxury can I give myself permission to enjoy today?

WHOLE-SELF CHECKLIST
- EXERCISE
- MEAL PLAN
- ALONE TIME
- SPIRITUAL INPUT
- SCHEDULED TIME TO PROCESS AN EXPERIENCE/FEELING

TOPIC	FORMAT	SOURCE

FAVORITE FACT:

I DON'T NEED TO HAVE **ALL THE ANSWERS** TO JOIN THE **CONVERSATION**

TODAY'S DATE

TODAY'S GOAL

TODAY'S EXPLORATIONS	GIVES ENERGY	NEUTRAL	TAKES ENERGY

T A S K S

MUST DO THIS WEEK

What is one step I can take to better my health?

Have I put up any walls? Is there anyone I need to forgive?

What luxury can I give myself permission to enjoy today?

WHOLE-SELF
C H E C K L I S T
- EXERCISE
- MEAL PLAN
- ALONE TIME
- SPIRITUAL INPUT
- SCHEDULED TIME TO PROCESS AN EXPERIENCE/FEELING

TOPIC	FORMAT	SOURCE

FAVORITE FACT:

I DON'T NEED TO HAVE **ALL THE ANSWERS** TO JOIN THE **CONVERSATION**

TODAY'S DATE

TODAY'S GOAL

TODAY'S EXPLORATIONS	GIVES ENERGY	NEUTRAL	TAKES ENERGY

T A S K S

MUST DO THIS WEEK

What is one step I can take to better my health?

Have I put up any walls? Is there anyone I need to forgive?

What luxury can I give myself permission to enjoy today?

WHOLE-SELF CHECKLIST
- EXERCISE
- MEAL PLAN
- ALONE TIME
- SPIRITUAL INPUT
- SCHEDULED TIME TO PROCESS AN EXPERIENCE/FEELING

TOPIC	FORMAT	SOURCE

FAVORITE FACT:

I DON'T NEED TO HAVE **ALL THE ANSWERS** TO JOIN THE **CONVERSATION**

TODAY'S DATE | **TODAY'S** GOAL

TODAY'S EXPLORATIONS	GIVES ENERGY	NEUTRAL	TAKES ENERGY	**T A S K S**

MUST DO THIS WEEK

What is one step I can take to better my health?

Have I put up any walls? Is there anyone I need to forgive?

What luxury can I give myself permission to enjoy today?

WHOLE-SELF CHECKLIST
- EXERCISE
- MEAL PLAN
- ALONE TIME
- SPIRITUAL INPUT
- SCHEDULED TIME TO PROCESS AN EXPERIENCE/FEELING

TOPIC	FORMAT	SOURCE

FAVORITE FACT:

I DON'T NEED TO HAVE **ALL THE ANSWERS** TO JOIN THE **CONVERSATION**

TODAY'S DATE

TODAY'S GOAL

TODAY'S EXPLORATIONS	GIVES ENERGY	NEUTRAL	TAKES ENERGY

T A S K S

MUST DO THIS WEEK

What is one step I can take to better my health?

Have I put up any walls? Is there anyone I need to forgive?

What luxury can I give myself permission to enjoy today?

WHOLE-SELF CHECKLIST
- EXERCISE
- MEAL PLAN
- ALONE TIME
- SPIRITUAL INPUT
- SCHEDULED TIME TO PROCESS AN EXPERIENCE/FEELING

TOPIC	FORMAT	SOURCE

FAVORITE FACT:

I DON'T NEED TO HAVE **ALL THE ANSWERS** TO JOIN THE **CONVERSATION**

TODAY'S DATE					**TODAY'S** GOAL

TODAY'S EXPLORATIONS	GIVES ENERGY	NEUTRAL	TAKES ENERGY	**T A S K S**

MUST DO THIS WEEK

What is one step I can take to better my health?

Have I put up any walls? Is there anyone I need to forgive?

What luxury can I give myself permission to enjoy today?

WHOLE-SELF CHECKLIST
- EXERCISE
- MEAL PLAN
- ALONE TIME
- SPIRITUAL INPUT
- SCHEDULED TIME TO PROCESS AN EXPERIENCE/FEELING

TOPIC	FORMAT	SOURCE

FAVORITE FACT:

I DON'T NEED TO HAVE **ALL THE ANSWERS** TO JOIN THE **CONVERSATION**

TODAY'S DATE | **TODAY'S** GOAL

TODAY'S EXPLORATIONS	GIVES ENERGY	NEUTRAL	TAKES ENERGY	T A S K S

MUST DO THIS WEEK

What is one step I can take to better my health?

Have I put up any walls? Is there anyone I need to forgive?

What luxury can I give myself permission to enjoy today?

WHOLE-SELF CHECKLIST
- EXERCISE
- MEAL PLAN
- ALONE TIME
- SPIRITUAL INPUT
- SCHEDULED TIME TO PROCESS AN EXPERIENCE/FEELING

TOPIC	FORMAT	SOURCE

FAVORITE FACT:

I DON'T NEED TO HAVE **ALL THE ANSWERS** TO JOIN THE **CONVERSATION**

TODAY'S DATE | **TODAY'S** GOAL

TODAY'S EXPLORATIONS	GIVES ENERGY	NEUTRAL	TAKES ENERGY	T	A	S	K	S

MUST DO THIS WEEK

What is one step I can take to better my health?

Have I put up any walls? Is there anyone I need to forgive?

What luxury can I give myself permission to enjoy today?

WHOLE-SELF CHECKLIST
- EXERCISE
- MEAL PLAN
- ALONE TIME
- SPIRITUAL INPUT
- SCHEDULED TIME TO PROCESS AN EXPERIENCE/FEELING

TOPIC	FORMAT	SOURCE

FAVORITE FACT.

I DON'T NEED TO HAVE **ALL THE ANSWERS** TO JOIN THE **CONVERSATION**

TODAY'S DATE

TODAY'S GOAL

TODAY'S EXPLORATIONS	GIVES ENERGY	NEUTRAL	TAKES ENERGY

T A S K S

MUST DO THIS WEEK

What is one step I can take to better my health?

Have I put up any walls? Is there anyone I need to forgive?

What luxury can I give myself permission to enjoy today?

WHOLE-SELF
C H E C K L I S T
- EXERCISE
- MEAL PLAN
- ALONE TIME
- SPIRITUAL INPUT
- SCHEDULED TIME TO PROCESS AN EXPERIENCE/FEELING

TOPIC

FORMAT

SOURCE

FAVORITE FACT:

I DON'T NEED TO HAVE **ALL THE ANSWERS** TO JOIN THE **CONVERSATION**

TODAY'S DATE   **TODAY'S** GOAL

TODAY'S EXPLORATIONS	GIVES ENERGY	NEUTRAL	TAKES ENERGY	**T A S K S**	

MUST DO THIS WEEK

What is one step I can take to better my health?

Have I put up any walls? Is there anyone I need to forgive?

What luxury can I give myself permission to enjoy today?

WHOLE-SELF CHECKLIST
- EXERCISE
- MEAL PLAN
- ALONE TIME
- SPIRITUAL INPUT
- SCHEDULED TIME TO PROCESS AN EXPERIENCE/FEELING

TOPIC	FORMAT	SOURCE

FAVORITE FACT:

I DON'T NEED TO HAVE **ALL THE ANSWERS** TO JOIN THE **CONVERSATION**

TODAY'S DATE | **TODAY'S** GOAL

TODAY'S EXPLORATIONS	GIVES ENERGY	NEUTRAL	TAKES ENERGY	**T A S K S**

MUST DO THIS WEEK

What is one step I can take to better my health?

Have I put up any walls? Is there anyone I need to forgive?

What luxury can I give myself permission to enjoy today?

WHOLE-SELF CHECKLIST
- EXERCISE
- MEAL PLAN
- ALONE TIME
- SPIRITUAL INPUT
- SCHEDULED TIME TO PROCESS AN EXPERIENCE/FEELING

TOPIC	FORMAT	SOURCE

FAVORITE FACT:

CPSIA information can be obtained
at www.ICGtesting.com
Printed in the USA
LVHW072103060121
675853LV00025B/1321